ABUSED (~~IRRITABLE~~) BOWEL SYNDROME:

WHAT CAUSES IBS AND WHAT TO DO ABOUT IT

notionpress.com

Abused (~~Irritable~~)
Bowel Syndrome:
What causes IBS and What To Do About It

Vikas Khurana, MD, MBA

notionpress.com

Notion Press

Copyright © Vikas Khurana, MD, United States of America, 2013
All Right Reserved.

First Print edition by Notion Press 2013
ISBN: 978-1-940955-00-1
Library of Congress Control Number: 2014903374

Doctors says: **"you have Irritable Bowel Syndrome (IBS)"**
Patients hears: **"you can't be helped".**

Why Should You Read This Book?

If you or a loved one has suffered from Irritable Bowel Syndrome, you will understand why the gut is one of the most important organs in your body and any malfunction of this organ can lead to severe anxiety, discomfort and sometimes depression.

There is a large group of patients who continue to suffer and search for the cause of their Irritable Bowel Syndrome. Their symptoms have been classified and sub-classified but the majority of them are provided no relief. They are given just another name which is used to explain their symptom complex. Treatments that work for one patient do not affect another. Patients are made to believe the next big thing is right around the corner and this goes on for years. Their symptoms continue to occur even after trying multiple medications, procedures, imaging, and even surgery.

Here's Not Just 1, but 9 Reasons Why:

1. If you wish to know more about why and how your bowel acts up during Irritable Bowel Syndrome and how your bowel function changes in health and disease.

2. If you have chronic recurrent abdominal pain which remains unexplained even after extensive medical evaluation and it was labeled Irritable Bowel Syndrome and you are asked to live with it.

3. If you have been given a diagnosis of Irritable Bowel Syndrome and want to understand why your symptoms are not under control even when you are following everything your doctor asked you to do.

4. If you used to get abdominal pain with constipation before and now you suffer from Diarrhea, and are consequently locked inside your house due to fear of soiling.

5. If you have tightness in the stomach, bloating, or back pain and people have convinced you that it's all in your head.

6. If you have occasional nausea and vomiting, dizziness, and stomach cramps. You tried fiber supplements and it made the symptoms worse.

7. If your bowel symptoms are confusing and you do not know where to start the discussion with your doctor or you feel ashamed to talk to your physician again.

8. If you have tried multiple recipes and treatments suggested by friends, family, and physicians and nothing has worked.

9. If you had the symptoms since childhood and all your hopes of getting better have been eliminated

---

This book gives you REAL answers that can stop your suffering. The solution to your symptoms is a LOT simpler than you thought. This book provides you with an understanding of Irritable Bowel Syndrome in simple language and arms you with the knowledge you need to tame Irritable Bowel Syndrome. It's time to get the relief you deserve.

About the Author

Vikas Khurana, MD, MBA

Dr Khurana is **board certified** by the **American Board of Internal Medicine** in Internal Medicine and Gastroenterology. He did his medical school from Maulana Azad Medical College in India, his residency in Internal Medicine from State University of New York at Brooklyn, New York, and his Gastroenterology fellowship from the University of Miami School of Medicine, Florida. He is a former **Associate Professor** of Medicine at Temple University, PA and Assistant Professor of Medicine and Computer Sciences at Louisiana State University. He also holds a Master of Business Administration from the Wharton Business School, University of Pennsylvania.

Dr. Khurana is a rare breed of clinician and researcher who continues to practice medicine and has rich clinical experience in treating gastro-intestinal ailments. He has taught and **trained doctors** in the field of gastroenterology at academic medical centers.

His first **research award** was in 1991 when he was in medical school and since then has received multiple research awards including the American College of Gastroenterology's National Governor's Award for Excellence in Clinical Research. He has received awards and presented his research at national meetings in various societies including the ACG, AGA and AASLD. At Wharton, Dr. Khurana received the Snider Seed Award for his project in healthcare. His research work has been cited in **Wall Street Journal, Forbes and USA today**. He has Supervised NIH and National VA studies and has numerous scientific journal articles, review articles and scientific presentations to his credit.

Dr. Khurana's work has been featured in interviews on **CNN, ABC and NBC.**

Dr. Khurana has been elected to several prestigious societies including **Alpha Omega Alpha (AOA)** Honor Medical Society and the Bokus International Gastroenterological Society. He was elected as a Fellow of American college of Gastroenterology (**FACG**), and a Fellow of the American college of Physicians (**FACP**).

The Facts

Insights are instantaneous and happen when all the dots connect; not all insights require million-dollar research. The facts below have changed and continue to change our understanding of Irritable Bowel Syndrome:

1. Pain does not happen to torture you, but rather acts as an early warning system to diagnose dysfunction and to bring it to your attention.

2. The colon is an active organ (not a passive tube) which moves the stool efficiently. It has the capacity to correct some (not all) of its dysfunctions.

3. Constipation comes first, and the rest of the symptoms follow in a predictable manner.

4. If the constipation is ignored, the body is not going to let the person die and will act to correct the constipation by secreting fluids and electrolytes to correct constipation, which is interpreted as diarrhea.

5. Different sections of the colon can have different problems at any given time.

6. Hydration of the body requires both water and electrolytes.

7. If constipation is prevented and the old residual stool flushed out, symptoms associated with IBS disappear.

Letter from the Doctor

Chronic recurrent abdominal pain is nothing new; we have known about this pain for over hundred years or more. Why can't we figure this disease out? We spend millions of dollars and all we do is suffer. We lose productive time and sufferers are labeled as a type of personality. People make fun of patients with IBS and colleagues treat them as social outcasts. There is no help given to them from the medical community. Are doctors unable to help? Is science impotent against this disease? Why are these people sentenced to suffer for life? Or is it that we never understood the disease well enough? In our quest to explain the bowel dysfunction we went too deep inside the jungle that we lost the big picture. We know more about the structure of colon cells than what the colon contains and how the stool moves around in the colon.

Over the last 15 years of my medical practice I have been perplexed and distressed by the sheer number of patients who continue to suffer from Irritable Bowel Syndrome even after an extensive medical workup. Patients are so confused that they don't want to tell the doctor where exactly the pain is, as it is everywhere and the doctors do not have any answers. This forced me to question *why*? As I learned from my mentors and the current textbooks, I realized the limitations of the current thought-process. I was encouraged by my mentors to ask questions and think outside the box and even though my mentors did not have answers for all my questions, they showed me the path. Once I graduated the structured curriculum, I started exploring. Irritable Bowel Syndrome is nothing new; humans have suffered from symptoms similar to Irritable Bowel Syndrome since we came into existence. This thought prompted me to explore the medical archives and literature that are over one thousand years old for similar conditions and their respective solutions. Even though clinicians in the last millennium did not have our technologies available to them, they had time and patience. They made observations and clinical correlations that were far superior to anything being described now. Suffering from recurrent chronic abdominal pain was nothing new and was not killing the patients but was a recurrent painful phase that these patients suffered from. Learning from those descriptions and adding on the modern technology and imaging a brand-new insight started developing in such disorders. The same patients I once feared the most taught me more than I could have ever imagined. They started teaching me new theories that forced me to go back to the basics in medicine. Suddenly things started to make sense. *Voila*, I hit the jackpot. The patients' symptoms started making physiological sense and their symptoms started getting better when treated with these new insights. My business training taught me to be consumer-oriented, realistic, and to question every assumption. Yet my medical training taught me to hold on to the defined conditions—the two philosophies collided and complemented each other to provide well-rounded inferences.

This book makes a humble effort in correcting this void. In my research I feel indebted to physicians and mentors from the past whose work had been preserved and made available due to modern technology. These include: Aretaeus of Cappadocia, Ayurveda literature (multiple authors), Thomas L. Brunton, MD; Henry M Field, M.D., William Arbuthnot-Lane, MS; Henry L. Bockus, MD, Arthur F. Hurst, MD, Jamie S Barkin, MD, Premashis Kar, MD and several others. With a noble intent driven by my desire to provide solutions to despairing patients,, I humbly share this information with the extensive readership.

Contents

Section 1: The Label of Irritable Bowel Syndrome

SPOTLIGHT ON

- Why and how your bowel acts up during Irritable Bowel Syndrome in simple language.

- Chronic recurrent abdominal pain which remains unexplained after investigations and was labeled Irritable Bowel Syndrome

"Irritable Bowel Syndrome" is one of the most commonly diagnosed conditions that has become the waste-paper diagnosis for abdominal pain. If the patient presents with abdominal pain, nausea, dizziness, anxiety, clay-like stools three to six times a day, and the known workup including upper endoscopy, colonoscopy, CT scans, abdominal X-rays, capsule endoscopy, stool or blood tests do not explain these symptoms, it is labeled as "Irritable Bowel Syndrome" or IBS. The fact remains that billions of dollars have been spent in search of a magic cure for this condition without much success. Many of the patients suffering from unexplained gastrointestinal symptoms were labeled as Irritable Bowel Syndrome during at least some period of their life.

I have also noticed that people who used to get constipation and have used a laxative believe that they can outgrow their constipation. Constipation is both self-treated and also treated by doctors. However, doctors have limited time now so patients are left to fend for themselves. There are definitely some kinds of constipation that are episodic and are related to medications and other reasons. Most often constipation is *idiopathic* (without a known reason), which is idiotic for the doctors and pathetic for the patients. It is idiotic because we cannot find a real cause, and pathetic because patients continue to suffer. For those taking medications that cause constipation, it is likely they will continue to need the medications for the long-term. I have seen many patients who were prescribed a medication with constipation as a side effect, and then forgot about it. As constipation grows slowly and the last week's picture of our health becomes the baseline of our health picture for next week, constipation is ignored and forgotten. People try to connect their symptoms with what they ate, yet this link is difficult to establish due to slow development of their symptoms and the food reaction may not be visible right away or even for few days.

Human memory for diet does not span for more than a few days. If the symptoms do not occur within twenty four hours of eating food, people do not relate their symptoms with their diet. Still, people will try to explain their symptoms based on what they ate. How can our brain comprehend that the constipation we are suffering from today is the result of what we ate three days or even a week ago? The relationship of food and symptoms becomes confusing as bowel upset may indeed be related to the food taken few days ago. The result is that people end up with unexplained abdominal pain, nausea and heartburn-like symptoms.

To be fair to patients and health professionals, unlike other ailments, the symptoms in constipation are often concealed and difficult to verbalize. Almost all findings are based on patient's experience of pain or nonspecific symptoms. Correlating the relationship between patient's symptom and his or her disease process is difficult. Add to that the time and pressure on the health provider and non-critical nature of the bowel disease. The result is that healthcare providers have stopped listening to patients and are too quick to label patients with a diagnosis.

I feel that the art of prevention and advice for lifestyle changes is vanishing from medical assessment. Doctors are under pressure to see too many patients and hence too busy to talk about constipation. Healthcare providers have a mental hierarchy and priority for symptoms and diseases, and the result is that constipation is left for the patients to manage themselves. This book helps patients understand the disease process better and provides them with information to manage their disease better. The book is for those patients who are too embarrassed to talk about this topic and sometimes ignored and hence continue to suffer.

Section 2: Pain and Irritable Bowel Syndrome

SPOTLIGHT ON

- Your pain is your body's warning system
- You **don't** have to suffer forever!
- Clinical Story: Could this be YOU?

What is Irritable Bowel Syndrome (IBS) in medical terms?

Irritable Bowel Syndrome (IBS) is a disorder caused by changes in how the digestive tract works. IBS is not a disease; it is a group of symptoms that occur together. The most common symptoms of IBS are abdominal pain or discomfort, often reported as cramping, along with diarrhea, constipation or both. IBS is diagnosed when a person has abdominal pain or discomfort at least three times per month for the last 3 months without any other disease or injury that could explain the pain. The pain or discomfort of IBS may occur with a change in stool frequency or consistency or may be relieved by a bowel movement. IBS is considered a functional gastrointestinal (GI) or digestive disorder. These people with a functional digestive disorder have frequent symptoms, but the digestive tract does not become permanently damaged. IBS is often classified into subtypes based on a person's usual stool consistency. The symptoms of IBS are abdominal pain or discomfort and changes in bowel habits. To meet the definition of IBS, the pain or discomfort should be associated with two of the following three symptoms:

- ⊙ Pain starts with bowel movements that occur more or less often than usual
- ⊙ Pain with stool that appears looser and more watery or harder and more lumpy than usual

- ⊙ Improvement with a bowel movement

Other symptoms of IBS may include:

- ⊙ Diarrhea—having loose, watery stools three or more times a day and feeling urgency to have a bowel movement

- ⊙ Constipation—having hard, dry stools; three or fewer bowel movements in a week; or straining to have a bowel movement

- ⊙ Feeling that a bowel movement is incomplete

- ⊙ Passing mucus, a clear liquid made by the intestines that coats and protects tissues in the digestive tract

- ⊙ Abdominal bloating

Symptoms may often occur after eating a meal. To meet the definition of IBS, symptoms must occur at least 3 days a month.

> I recommend every patient visit the following site to get complete medical information on IBS: http://digestive.niddk. nih.gov/ddiseases/pubs/ibs

Why do we experience pain in IBS?

Pain is a text message to your brain that something is wrong with the body system—just like a fire alarm it is a call to attention. When the fire alarm goes off, we can respond by putting on earmuffs or taking the battery out, or we can extinguish the fire or we can run. Ignoring the fire alarm will not prevent us from getting burnt. Similarly, the symptoms change and health problems escalate if initial call to attention is ignored.

Clinical Story

I have had Irritable Bowel Syndrome for a long time and my doctors convinced me that I have to suffer...

A 36-year-old lady came for an evaluation because of cramping and abdominal pain, which had been ongoing for several years.

She had seen several doctors for her pain and was diagnosed with diarrhea predominant Irritable Bowel Syndrome. Once she was diagnosed with IBS, her doctor remarked that she couldn't do much about her pain and therefore must bear it. She had abdominal pain in a band-like fashion radiating from the right upper side to the left upper side of her abdomen. She also complained of feeling dizzy, weak, having hot and cold flashes, and having the feeling of fainting. She had pain in her lower left abdomen with cramping. Her bowel movement pattern was unusual. She used to get six to eight bowel movements per day. However, she occasionally got constipated for an entire week. She also complained of having bowel movements after every meal and she experienced a plugged sensation, which she described as the "cork in wine bottle" sensation where the first piece of stool was hard to pass, after which the stool flowed smoothly. She was prescribed fiber but her symptoms got worse whenever she took fiber supplements. In her words she felt as if she was "adding more fuel to the fire". The patient subsequently underwent an upper endoscopy and a colonoscopy to rule out any organic disease process and both were negative. No ulcers were found and no microscopic colitis was found on random colonic biopsies.

Interestingly, after the colonoscopy her symptoms went away and she was symptom-free for a few days, after which the symptoms came back gradually and she was having all the symptoms by two weeks. Given the response to cleaning her colon, she was prescribed laxatives and acid suppression which caused significant relief of symptoms. The symptoms did not go away completely but were more manageable and predictable.

> **Lesson Learned:** Constipation is a significant component of Irritable Bowel Syndrome and I believe it is the initiator of the cycle of Irritable Bowel Syndrome. If the pain pattern changes after taking preparation for a colonoscopy and returns back to baseline in a few days to weeks, constipation should be strongly considered. An attempt of laxative use should be considered in collaboration with your healthcare provider.

Section 3: Lifecycle of Irritable Bowel Syndrome

SPOTLIGHT ON

- Importance of the gut
- Understanding the Digestive Tract and how it relates to IBS
- Lifecycle of IBS

What is the Colon?

The digestive system is a 20-40 feet long tube that starts at the throat and ends at the anus. The tube is responsible for passing the food that we eat as well as extracting all the nutrients we need. The residual material is passed as stool. The food enters the mouth and travels through the esophagus, stomach, small intestine, and large intestine and exits the anus as stool. Each segment of this tube is controlled by entry and exit valves called sphincters. Except for eating and the passage of stool the entire process is automated and occurs at a subconscious level.

The digestion and absorption of the nutrients occurs primarily in the small intestine. The residual food material along with shedding of dead cells and secretions of liver and pancreas are passed on to the colon. *Peristalsis*, or slow contractile muscular activity, helps to propel the undigested food towards the anus and allows the food to be excreted. The Colon is five feet long, and what is excreted as stool is the result of the last one to two feet of the colon. The functioning or malfunctioning of the other four feet is not visible to us. Unfortunately, it is assumed that the entire colon function is represented by the stool that is passed.

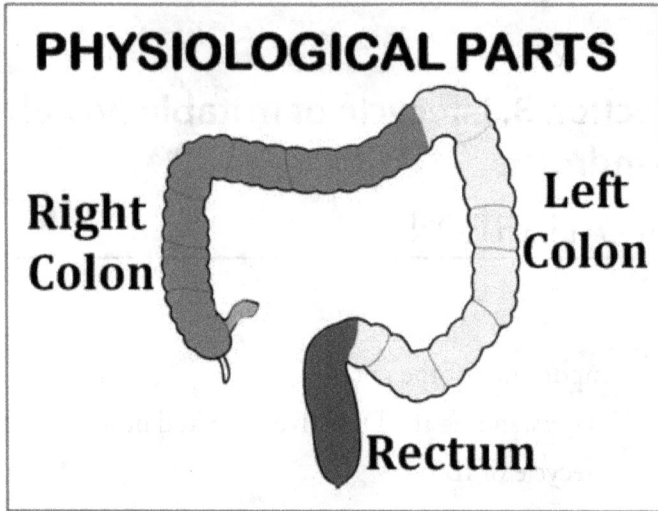

Figure 1   Physiological Parts of the Colon

The process of fluid and electrolyte absorption starts in the cecum and continues in the ascending and transverse colon. The cecum is distensible which permits storage of large volumes of semi-liquid stool that enters from the small bowel. The right side of the colon is responsible for absorption, and the left side of the colon is responsible for the storage of stool. The stool consistency changes from mostly liquid in the cecum and ascending colon to thick paste in the transverse colon, semisolid in the descending colon and to solid stool in the sigmoid colon. Normally the right side of the colon is devoid of any solid stool (liquid stool is present but no solid stool should be present). Most of the time, the rectum is empty of feces. Normally the stool should stay soft until defecated. If the person is dehydrated or if stool stays in contact with colonic mucosa for long, water is removed from the stool which makes it hard.

Over the last one hundred years, extensive research has been done to prove that the colon is not a passive tube through which the stool passes. Rather, it encompasses several functions which are very important for the survival of humans. These functions not only include absorption of fluids and electrolytes, but also secretion of electrolytes and mucous to lubricate the stool. Functionally the three major segments of the colon are:

1. The right side of the colon which is involved with absorption of water, electrolytes, and some nutrients from the undigested food, and helps in changing the consistency of stool from liquid to semisolid stool.

2. The left side of the colon, which is involved with storage of stool until it can be expelled.

3. The rectum, which is involved with the controlled excretion of the stool.

The principal functions of the colon are: absorption of water, absorption of salt, and the storage of stool until it can be expelled. The movements of the colon are slow but well-orchestrated and provide two functions: mixing the stool and moving the stool towards the anus to be expelled from the body. When colonic movement forces stool into the rectum, the desire for defecation occurs. When it becomes convenient for the person to defecate, there is contraction of the rectum and relaxation of the anal sphincters resulting in defecation or passage of stool.

Life Cycle of Irritable Bowel Syndrome

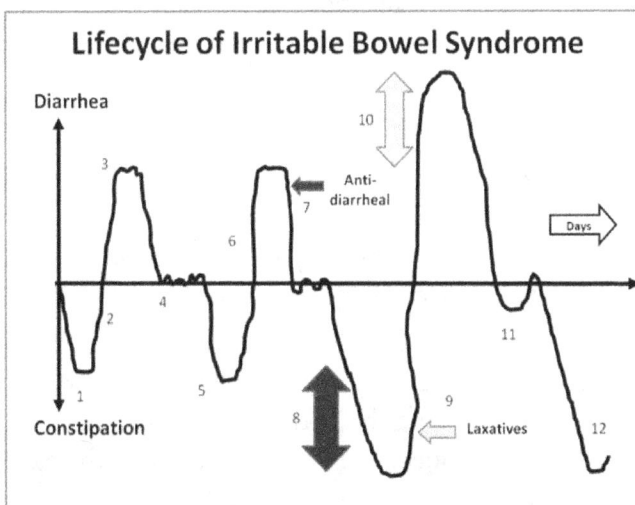

Figure 2   Life Cycle of Irritable Bowel Syndrome

1. The initial precipitating factor might be excessive sweating, not drinking water, travel, excessive caffeine or any other cause which might dehydrate a person. With dehydration, excess water is removed from the stool and the stool is hardened. The first piece of stool is the hardest to pass and if the patient is unable to pass the hard stool in a timely fashion, constipation starts.

2. This is followed by body's corrective response to severe constipation which is secretion of potassium and bicarbonate-rich fluid in the distal colon to dissolve the impacted stool. This is interpreted as loose bowel by the patient.

3. Patient may get multiple loose bowel movements at this stage.

4. A few good days without symptoms follow the bout of loose bowels, during which the patient may not have or constipation or loose bowel.

5. Another slew of precipitating factors will cause another episode of constipation and worsening constipation for a few days. Symptoms are easily ignored at this stage as Patients get more time to do other things! Severe constipation that causes retention of stool and the stool becomes harder and more difficult to pass.

6. Again this is followed by loose bowel movements. It may be reported as diarrhea by patients and they waste time sitting on the toilet.

7. Patients generally pay more attention to diarrhea, as it limits the mobility and interferes with their lifestyle. To correct symptoms anti-diarrheal medication is taken.

8. The anti-diarrheal medication works for that day, but by this time the body's corrective action has stopped and the medicine further constipates the patient.

9. As the constipation becomes severe, abdominal pain starts which cannot be ignored. People search for

a cause and notice constipation to be the culprit. In search for relief they take a dose of laxative correct the severe constipation..

10. By the time laxatives take effect, the patient has already moved from the constipation phase to normal due to the corrective response of the body which is secreting fluids and electrolytes. The laxatives cause exacerbation of the next cycle of diarrhea.

11. The patient is thoroughly confused by this cycle and seeks medical help. Constipation and diarrhea continue to occur and patients undergo extensive workup to rule out organic diseases. Once the workup is negative, the diagnosis of Irritable Bowel Syndrome is made. They are told take laxatives when constipated and antidiarrheal when having diarrhea.

12. And the cycle continues with wide variations of bowel habits.

Patients continue to suffer and once the label of Irritable Bowel Syndrome is given, they are made to believe that they have to suffer. The only help is to correct their constipation with laxatives and diarrhea with anti-diarrheal medication. Advice regarding modification of diet, stress and other factors is given, which is more easily prescribed than done. Internet and health literature is loaded with anecdotal information about what worked and what did not work, confusing patients further. Some of these suggestions or medications may help if they address the precipitating constipation. Many patients will continue to get increasingly worse with fewer healthy days and will hope for a new drug that will be approved for this condition.

Section 4: Constipation and Irritable Bowel Syndrome
SPOTLIGHT ON

---

* Abdominal pain with constipation before and now diarrhea
* Tightness in the stomach, bloating, or back pain
* Occasional nausea and vomiting, dizziness, and stomach cramps

The book makes no claims to *cure* most of Irritable Bowel Syndrome by treating bowel irregularities but *understanding* this disease will make the lives of these patients with IBS more manageable. Over the last several years, Irritable Bowel Syndrome has perplexed me. It is because patients continue to suffer, and there are not many treatment options available. This makes me as a physician uncomfortable. We as a medical community were unable to explain why patients undergo pain, why they have diarrhea-predominant or constipation-predominant symptoms, and what the common thread throughout this tapestry is. As I started to investigate, it became clear that this condition has existed for a few generations and has been researched extensively by the previous generations. Previous generations lacked the scientific tools but they did have strong analytical and observational skills. Current medicine has taken a very different scientific direction— namely too much emphasis on statistical numbers. Having been involved with these studies, I have realized that rigorous design and randomized research trials return important results but sometimes we lose the main focus while conducting these long-term and extremely costly studies. Irritable Bowel Syndrome, like many other medical problems, does not occur in isolation.

Over years of discussions with patients and through my own critical evaluation of medical literature, it has dawned on me that IBS is just an extension of constipation in many patients. There are pain perception issues that have been extensively researched and the modification of pain perception provides significant relief to select patients. However, the underlying constipation is generally not treated. There are several assumptions we make that prevent us from effectively treating Irritable Bowel Syndrome-like symptoms. I do believe in the outstanding research being done to develop therapies for Irritable Bowel Syndrome. They have made definite strides in treating this highly perplexing disease. *However most of the patients labeled with Irritable Bowel Syndrome are in fact suffering from a less exotic term—constipation.* Randomized double-blind, placebo-controlled trials have shown that medications which improve the motility of the colon are effective in the treatment of patients with constipation predominant Irritable Bowel Syndrome (Novick 2002). Recently, the same medication has been shown to improve symptoms for patients with mixed (diarrhea and constipation) Irritable Bowel Syndrome (Cehy, 2008). In spite of these advances, patients continue to suffer and millions of dollars are being spent to find a universal cure for IBS.

While talking to many patients with Irritable Bowel Syndrome it became clear that most of these patients suffer from constipation alternating with diarrhea. Their symptoms did get better after a colonoscopy preparation in which the entire stool-load of the colon is removed to perform visual inspection. Furthermore, the symptoms come back within few weeks. It has been shown that by inflating a balloon in the colon, abdominal pain similar to the pain encountered by patients with Irritable Bowel Syndrome can be reproduced. (Ritche, 1973 and Swarbrick, 1980) Similarly, the retained stool also causes distention, which is felt as pain or discomfort by the patients. These initial observations in combination with experimental and clinical data made me question the diagnosis of Irritable Bowel Syndrome in a large number of patients. I started treating patients of the so-called

Irritable Bowel Syndrome with laxatives and had excellent results in most. Obviously not everyone responded but the majority of them had symptom relief. Most IBS patients can tell that the best days are immediately after an episode of diarrhea. This led me to propose the **lifecycle** of Irritable Bowel Syndrome. Whether IBS is over-diagnosed in constipated patients or is an extension of constipation is to be defined by further research. .

Section 5: Ask-the-Doc

◆ Are your bowel habits confusing? The Doc helps you understand your symptoms, right here, right now.

Q. 1. **I was told that bowel movement once or twice a week is okay. Is this really true?**

Dr. Khurana says: Medical research studies show that a bowel movement between three times a day to three times a week is normal (Connell, 1965). This was further reinforced by additional studies (Drossman, 1982). However this does not apply to patients who are having symptoms of frequent abdominal pain or nausea. Another caveat in this study was that these patients were regularly having the SAME number of bowel movements. It is abnormal if the numbers of bowel movements are fluctuating from week to week and are associated with abdominal symptoms. In addition, for those patients who are regularly having less than three bowel movements a week and not complaining of symptoms, it might be okay for now but long-term complications relating to constipation may occur. Such patients can be classified as having **subclinical constipation**. A trial of dietary modification and lifestyle changes or an empiric trial of laxatives may be helpful to understand the baseline symptoms.

Q. 2. **I did not poop for few days because I did not eat much for the entire last week. That's normal, right?**

Dr. Khurana says: Wrong. The stool normally is composed of about 75% water and 25% solid matter. The solid component is about 30% dead bacteria, 10 to 20% fat, 10 to 20% inorganic matter, 2 to 3% protein, and 30% undigested roughage from the food, digestive juices and sloughed cells from the internal lining of the digestive tract. Even though ingested food is a major component, there are several other components of stool that do not require a person to eat. Patients with colostomy have their colon disconnected and anchored to the abdominal wall from where the stool is collected in a bag. These people still continue to have infrequent bowel movement through the anus even though no food is flowing through the colon.

Most of the patients, who do not get a bowel movement for few days and are complaining of abdominal symptoms, are constipated. Alternatively they have dilated colon which can retain significant amount of fecal matter before the urge to defecate occurs. It is important to note that the dilated colon is not seen in patients without constipation. *If not passing stool for few days is associated with symptoms or a change in symptoms, medical attention should be sought.*

Extensive work has been done to help us understand constipation and its associated symptoms. However, we are still unable to help patients suffering with constipation in a meaningful way. The reasons behind this are numerous and beyond the scope of this book. I believe a single misinterpretation of literature has led us to this state of affairs. In 1965 it was shown that normal people have between three bowel movements a day to three bowel movements a week. This literature was misinterpreted to mean that having three bowel movements a day or having three bowel movements a week or anything in between was normal. However it was totally ignored that this was valid only for people who were not having digestive tract symptoms and the number was for patients with a consistent defecation pattern as discussed above. This assumption did a disservice to uninformed patients as they, along with the doctors, no longer believed altered bowel habits to be a significant cause of abdominal pain and discomfort.

Statistically, normal humans have a much more simple and standard frequency of defecation not too far from once or twice daily, which generally is constant for healthy patients. However when you talk to a patient experiencing abdominal pain and constipation, it is evident that their symptoms are related to fluctuations in the number of bowel movements. Believing abdominal pain to be an entity that has to be tamed immediately was the second mistake. Taking narcotic pain medicine worsens the constipation and the symptoms. *Pain is our body's warning system* that will start sending a signal whenever there is something wrong and immediate attention is required to that area. Revisiting the concept with this frame of reference made it clear that patients with subclinical constipation who do not complain of constipation-related symptoms are in fact able to suppress this pain so as to block it from conscious memory. Subsequently, once constipation is initially ignored, it presented itself as a collected set of symptoms and complications. Lastly, due to increased focus on pain evaluation in compliance with regulatory guidance, narcotic prescriptions increased dramatically which further increased the development of constipation in patients.

Q 3.   I was diagnosed with Irritable Bowel Syndrome and the pain is there all the time. However, I experience constipation sometimes. How can you explain that?

Dr. Khurana says: The colon is five feet long; what we poop is the result of the last one feet of colon and the functions or malfunctioning of the other four feet is not visible to us. The hard stool that is passed is residing in the rectosigmoid (or the left side of the colon), while diarrhea and constipation is noticed based on the stool consistency on the left side of the colon. However if the stool on the right side gets hardened, we can still have soft stool in the left side causing diarrhea and hard stool on the right side of the colon causing pain.

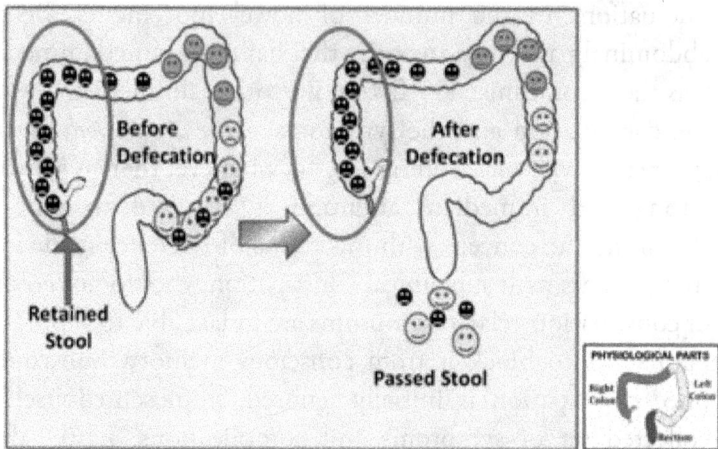

Figure 3   Retained Stool in the Right Colon

As seen above, even though the stool balls in the lower part of the colon were passed, the hard balls higher up remain, which causes pain and discomfort. This explains why retained stool on the right side of the colon can continue to cause symptoms in patients without classic constipation.

Q. 4.   I get pain relief on the left side after I poop but the pain on the right side worsens after I poop. How come this is happening?

Dr. Khurana says: This is not very uncommon but a very confusing symptom in patients. We have to understand that the colon does not work as a plastic tube in which food enters from one end and stool comes out of the other. Different parts of the colon can get constipated regardless of what is happening in the other side of the colon. In the example below, three different areas have solid stool which is impacted.

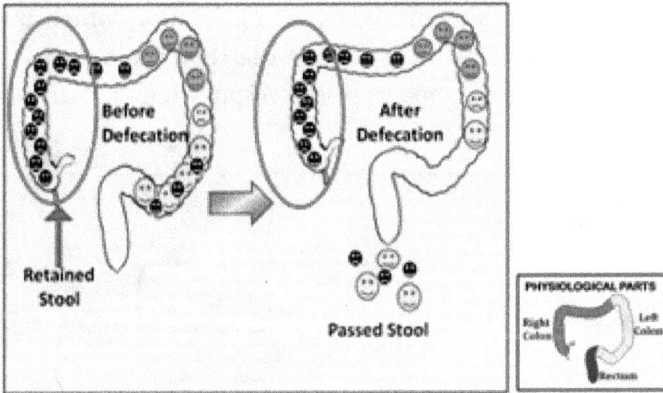

Figure 4   Stool Impaction in Different Segments of the Colon

In Figure 4, the stool in the left side of the colon was passed, causing the pain or discomfort to get better on the left side. However, stool on the right side of the colon is retained and the colon's attempt to move the stool on the right side causes pain and discomfort. Sometimes the stool on the right side of the colon is too large or too hard, or the muscle is relatively weak and the colon is not able to move the stool. The attempt to pass the stool on the right side causes colonic contractions, which is felt as cramping and abdominal pain.

Q. 5.   It is so confusing that constipation is presenting as diarrhea. How is it even possible?

Dr. Khurana says: The colon has a built-in protective response in case of its malfunction. Constipation when allowed to continue can worsen and lead to secretion of fluids and electrolytes as the body's defense mechanism to dissolve the hard-impacted stool. This secreted liquid flows around the hard balls of stool reaching the rectum rapidly. Once the fluid comes into the rectum an urge to defecate is stimulated. The urge becomes increasingly severe as more and more liquid stool enters the rectum, leading the patient to run to the bathroom. What is passed is liquid stool mixed with hard balls of stool. Since there is a significant amount of liquid stool, it is labeled as diarrhea. This confuses the patient.

Most patients take anti-diarrheal medication which makes the constipation worse. This causes diarrhea again and eventually diarrhea-troubled body stops responding to anti-diarrheal medications.

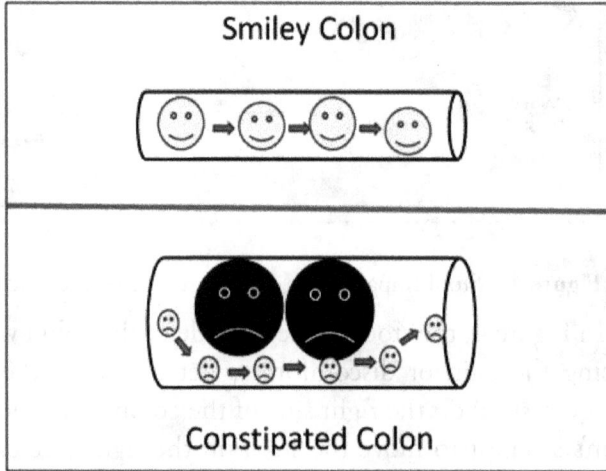

Figure 5   Healthy stool flow (top) and overflow diarrhea in colon with stool impaction (bottom)

To learn more about this phenomenon you need to understand the concept of congestive colon failure. Once the colon starts to fail it starts to dilate and when it is stretched beyond a limit it fails and cannot recover from it and becomes a passive failed tube which is a source of pain and suffering to many patients of ignored IBS.

Q. 6.   I get diarrhea every time I eat. Before, the anti-diarrheal medications were working, but now they do not. Why does this happen?

Dr. Khurana says: People who get constipated and ignore the constipation will eventually end up having "overflow diarrhea". Think of it like a river flow being blocked by rocks falling in its path. Eventually the water spills over the rock and starts flowing. Once the rock is removed the river size returns back to baseline. Similarly, the constipated hard stool blocks the flow of stool through the colon. Eventually the body's response is to make the stool liquid by secreting fluid and electrolytes which leads to the trickling of the fluid around the hard balls of stool, leading to diarrhea. *Yet the real problem was always constipation.* Once the patient is treated with laxatives and the hard balls of stool are removed, the symptoms return to baseline. Anti-diarrheal medications may exacerbate the symptoms by worsening the constipation and working against the corrective response of the body. Eventually, the body overcomes the effects of anti-diarrheal medication and it is no longer possible to control diarrhea with anti-diarrheal medications.

Q. 7.   My doctor gave me laxatives but instead of helping it worsened my pain and diarrhea. Why does this happen to me?

Dr. Khurana says: In some cases of congestive colon failure, the laxatives will move rapidly into the colon leading to the distention of the colon, causing worsening gas, cramps, and diarrhea. The laxatives can flow around the solid stool in cases of severe constipation and rapidly reach the rectum and cause diarrhea. Sometimes incomplete treatment is worse than no treatment because it irritates the disease state but does not cure it, leading to worsening symptoms. Hence it is important to take an adequate amount of laxatives to completely flush out all the constipated hard balls of stool. In case you are having significant abdominal pain which persists, stop the laxatives and discuss with your healthcare provider. In some cases of severe congestive colon failure, this can lead to fluid and electrolyte imbalance that can be life-threatening and should not be taken lightly. In case you are having significant diarrhea that persists, stop the laxatives and discuss with your healthcare provider.

Q. 8.   How long will it take for my bowel habits to return to normal?

Dr. Khurana says: That's a difficult question to answer as we're aware colon took different time **to distend with stool in different patients.** Not all distention of the colon will work in the same way. Think of it like dealing with an addict—give them one chance and he or she slips right back to old habits. We have to be religious with the bowel regimen and over weeks to months to years the colon will start shrinking and regain its normal size. However, no objective data for this is available at this point. The symptoms may not return to normal immediately and part of it can be explained by increased sensitivity of the body to normal physiological activities of the bowel. Some symptoms may be pathological and require pain altering medication including psychiatric medications. The pain definitely improves after flushing the colon and the symptoms of nausea, vomiting, diarrhea and poor appetite are generally resolved. The goal is to be consistent in the bowel regimen and **not let the colon get distended** with solid stool. The distention of colon due to the collection of solid stool has to be flushed to prevent the return of the symptoms. Think of it like colonic training.

Q. 9.   My doctor gave me laxatives but it did not help the pain; instead it worsened my pain. Why does this happen to me?

Dr. Khurana says: In some cases of longstanding constipation, the laxatives will move rapidly into the colon leading to the distention of the colon which causes worsening gas, cramps and diarrhea. The laxatives can flow around the solid stool in cases of severe constipation and rapidly reach the rectum causing diarrhea (Figure 5). To understand this better think of it like a hunter going to the jungle with a stick and finding a tiger. Not comprehending the situation clearly, the hunter uses the stick to kill the tiger. The stick is not going to finish the job and will instead only irritate the tiger. Sometimes incomplete treatment is worse than no treatment because it irritates the disease state but does not cure it, which leads to worsening symptoms. Hence it is important to take an adequate amount of laxatives to completely flush out all the constipated hard balls of stool. In case you are having significant abdominal pain or diarrhea that persists, stop the laxatives and discuss with your healthcare provider.

Section 6: Diet and Irritable Bowel Syndrome
SPOTLIGHT ON

- Fiber supplements made the symptoms worse; what is the role of fiber?
- Having tried multiple suggested recipes and treatments but nothing has worked

Diet and IBS

There is an extensive amount of information regarding what to eat and what not to eat if you're suffering from Irritable Bowel Syndrome including: caffeine, high-fiber products, spices, fried food, multigrain breads, salads, cabbage, beans, lentils, artificial sweeteners, sorbitol, and many others. These products have been linked to the worsening of symptoms because many stimulate the colon and are recommended to treat or prevent constipation. Diets low in fiber like soy, rice, potatoes, white bread, meat, eggs, and limited quantity of fruits are recommended to help patients with Irritable Bowel Syndrome. These recommendations are derived from years of experience by patients with Irritable Bowel Syndrome who have told their doctors and have written about what has helped them while dealing with IBS. Even a celiac diet and no carbohydrate or fiber diets have been advised. Incidentally they do help, as they decrease the volume of stool present in the colon which improves the symptoms and gives temporary relief which people are too glad to announce to the world. When after a few weeks to months relief of such symptoms stops and the patients get pain again, they are too scared to admit their pain is back. They continue to suffer and keep finding dietary reasons to cure IBS. No wonder we have recipes and cookbooks for IBS which work but fall short of long-term relief. For this reason people continue their search for the magical fix.

Based on such experiences, an extensive list has been created to which most of the patients add more food items leading to highly restricted diet leading t o additional nutritional deficiencies.

Over the last several years I have treated several patients with the label of Irritable Bowel Syndrome who turn out to have poorly managed constipation. Understanding that constipation can present in various forms based on the severity and length was ignored. Irritable Bowel Syndrome or as I call Ignored Constipation Syndrome (ICS) generally resolves when the constipation is treated. It is important to understand that it is an analogous chicken or egg problem: what comes first, the constipation or the pain? Once constipation sets in, pain and suffering will follow. *The only way to avoid these cycles is to avoid getting constipated.*

Even though fiber is recommended for most patients with constipation, it does not work the same way for all patients. Many patients will get flatulence, bloating, worsening of constipation or abdominal pain with fiber supplements. If taking fiber supplements makes your symptoms worse, then hold off on fiber for a few days and restart with a lower dose and gradually build up to the required dose. It is important to note that the endpoint is to have no symptoms associated with constipation; in other words, the dose of fiber supplement is not the endpoint. The number and consistency of the bowel movements is what needs to be focused on, and the dose of the fiber supplement should be titrated to have one to two soft bowel movements a day.

How Fiber Works to Keep People Regular

As the stool moves from the right side to the left side the water is removed from the stool. Normally the stool should stay soft until defecated. If the person is dehydrated or if the stool stays in contact with colonic mucosa for long, water is removed from stool which makes it hard. As the water content of the stool decreases, the stool becomes harder and heavier to move around in the colon.

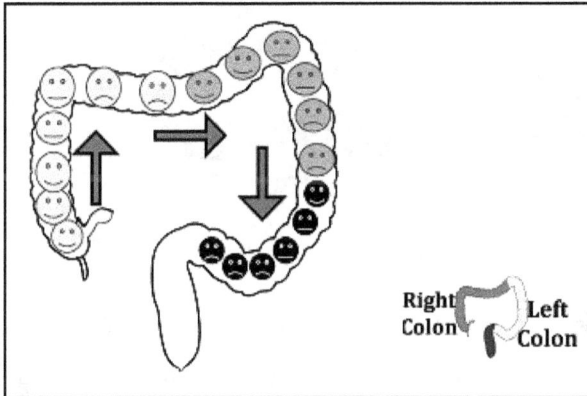

Figure 6   Water Absorption from the stool, the darker stool is harder and has less water and hence difficult to move

When people take fiber, the passage of the stool speeds up through the colon and less water is absorbed which leads to soft fluffy stool that is passed frequently. The essential requirement for fiber to work is that the colon should not be dilated and should function as a tube. The stool content needs to travel in one line. In a non-dilated colon the fiber works well and keeps the stool soft when passed. However, if the colon is dilated, which is the case with many people with long standing constipation; the fiber is counterproductive and causes further distention of the already-dilated colon leading to worsening of symptoms.

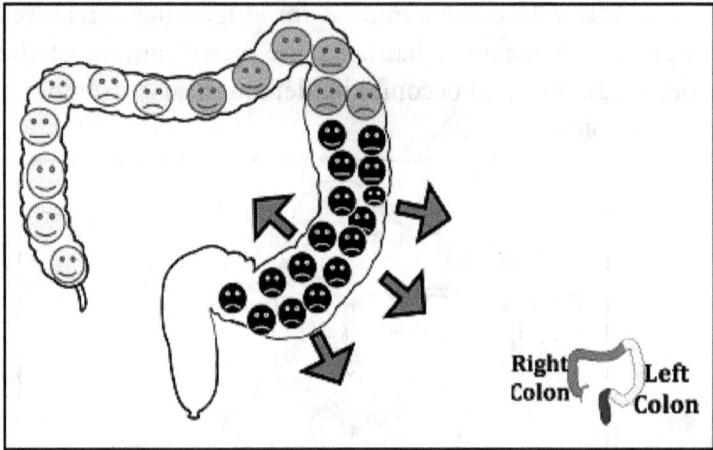

Figure 7 Colon Retails hard Stool and causes distention leading to pain

The symptoms of pain, nausea, and vomiting are mostly related to stool-causing distention of the colon. Passage of Hard stool will cause pain during defecation but a dilated distended colon with hard stool will cause constant symptoms even when no stool is being passed. Fiber adds more fuel to the fire and distends the colon further. Hence depending on the state of the colon fiber may or may not help the patient.

Section 7: Treatment of Irritable Bowel Syndrome

SPOTLIGHT ON

- Seven major treatment principles
- Bristol Stool Chart

Treatment of Irritable Bowel Syndrome

1. Flush the colon to remove all of the retained stool
2. Prevent the formation of hard stool
3. Correct the dehydration
4. Adjust diet to prevent constipation
5. Titrate laxatives
6. Incorporate physical activity and exercise
7. If all fails, repeat the flush and increase the laxative

1. Flush the Colon to Remove All of the Retained Stool

The first step to resolve the pain and symptoms of nausea, bloating, gas, and hard stool is to flush the entire content of the colon. This can be accomplished via multiple ways including over-the-counter laxatives, prescription laxatives which are used for colonoscopy preparation, or the use of colonic enemas. The goal is to remove the entire stool content of the colon. The rapidity of laxative intake is important during this process. If the laxative is taken slowly, it will flow around the hardened stool leading to diarrhea. Without the removal of hard stool, the symptoms will persist. One has to be careful and maintain a balance between the symptoms. The symptoms of abdominal distention, gas, and bloating will get worse when the laxatives start working on the colon. To prevent vomiting avoid ingesting any solid food prior to taking laxatives. This is best done early in the morning before taking any food. Most of the time if the laxatives are taken correctly the symptoms will be short-lived leading to long-term relief. It is important to take plenty of fluids and electrolytes. Patients with renal disease, heart disease, elderly patients, or patients with significant health problems should consult their doctor to find a safe laxative for their condition.

2. Prevent the Formation of Hard Stool

Patients will find relief from passing stool. However the relief is short-lived as the stool starts collecting and hardening again. To prevent the formation of hard stool again, long-term laxatives are recommended. An adequate dose of over-the-counter laxative or a prescription laxative is recommended to prevent the formation of hard stool. The type of laxative is important and should be an osmotic laxative or stool softener; the use of fiber is counterproductive at this stage. Stool softeners are milder form of laxatives and brand names include Colace, Docusate and Surfak. A variety of osmotic laxatives are available over-the-counter and as prescription. Some osmotic laxatives Brand names are Milk of Magnesia, Fleet Phospho-Soda, Cephulac, Sorbitol and MiraLax.

3. Titrate Laxatives

It is important to understand that the prescribed dose of laxative will rarely be the correct dose for the patient. The dose of laxative has to be adjusted to suit the individual patient. The goal is complete resolution of symptoms including abdominal pain, gas, nausea, bloating, or passage of hard stools.

To help understand the seven types of stool, please refer to chart below.

Bristol Stool Chart

Type 1		Separate hard lumps, like nuts (hard to pass)
Type 2		Sausage-shaped but lumpy
Type 3		Like a sausage but with cracks on the surface
Type 4		Like a sausage or snake, smooth and soft
Type 5		Soft blobs with clear-cut edges
Type 6		Fluffy pieces with ragged edges, a mushy stool
Type 7		Watery, no solid pieces. **Entirely Liquid**

As seen in the chart Types 1, 2, and 3 are hard constipated stool that will make the colon work harder than required. This causes symptoms to occur. Once you have suffered from symptoms of Irritable Bowel Syndrome these types of stool should always be avoided. Type 4 is too close to the constipated stool and should not be the target. The goal in patients with Irritable Bowel Syndrome should be to have between 1 to 3 soft stools per day of type 5 or type 6. If the stool is of type 7 and there are no associated symptoms the laxatives should be decreased. The goal is not the amount of laxative but rather to have one to three bowel movements a day and no symptoms. Titrating the laxatives to that goal is important and is done by increasing or decreasing the dose based on the type of stool in the above chart.

4. Correct Dehydration

Whenever a person is dehydrated there are two organs which conserve water: the kidneys and the colon. Once the kidney has reached its capacity to conserve water the colon starts removing water from the stool which leads to hardening of the stool. Prevention of dehydration is paramount in preventing the symptoms of Irritable Bowel Syndrome. Once the water is removed from the stool there is no way to add in water to the stool even if the person is well hydrated. Cyclical over-hydration and under-hydration does not mean normal hydration. The goal here is to have the urine color clear or light yellow and feel well hydrated. Passage of dark colored urine suggests that your body suffered an episode of dehydration. Mostly dehydration occurs when we sleep during the night. Water intake has to be balanced and avoid taking excess water before sleeping which may lead to disturbed sleep and waking up during the night to pee. A balance has to be maintained. The second part of dehydration is electrolyte balance. If the body is deficient of electrolyte and excess water is taken, the kidneys will throw the water out and lose additional body electrolytes in the process. This will further worsen the dehydration and symptoms. The correct thing to do in this situation is to take an electrolyte solution like Gatorade or a similar source of fluid containing high salt content. Patients with hypertension and other diseases which require low-salt consumption should be careful and should consult their doctor before taking electrolyte solution.

5. Adjust Diet to Prevent Constipation

A diet high in fresh fruits and vegetables will help the colon get adjusted to a normal healthy diet. As diet improves, the requirement of laxatives will decrease over time. The goal is to be off routine laxatives and only use them when constipation is predicted. This does not mean that the laxatives can be stopped immediately. It will take up to six months to a year before you can stop using laxatives. This will not happen in all cases and regular laxatives may be required for life. Further adjustment to one's diet may further decrease the laxative requirement.

6. Incorporate Physical Activity and Exercise

Physical activity and exercise is important to stimulate colonic motility. It becomes counterproductive if the person is dehydrated and the water is removed from the colon. Again, a balance has to be maintained when completing moderate physical activity and exercise without getting dehydrated. Adequate hydration with water alone or with electrolyte solution is helpful during vigorous exercise.

7. If All Fails, Repeat the Flush and Increase the Laxative

It is important to understand all is not lost when the titration of laxatives does not work. All it means is that the correct dose was not selected. Unfortunately we have to do the flush again and start the laxative at a higher dose and keep adjusting the dose of laxative. It is important to note that as the colon starts getting used to healthy stool it starts regaining strength and its functionality returns. This will be evident by the decreased requirement of laxative use.

In the end...

It is important to understand that not all abdominal symptoms are related to Irritable Bowel Syndrome. Just because a diagnosis of Irritable Bowel Syndrome was given to you, it does not mean that you will not get diseases that are common including colon cancer and colitis. Several patients with colon cancer and colitis will get a delayed diagnosis because their symptoms were attributed to Irritable Bowel Syndrome. Although this book suggests ways to test out the assumptions behind Irritable Bowel Syndrome it does not replace the careful and meticulous evaluation by a physician. Any new symptom should be investigated appropriately. **In the end I would like to say that *Abused Bowel Syndrome (ABS)* is more appropriate and meaningful term to define the symptoms of Irritable Bowel Syndrome. Once you abuse your bowels by ignoring constipation they will eventually cry out in pain and if the pain is ignored, additional symptoms will result. This has resulted in significant suffering and confusion for the patients with Irritable Bowel Syndrome.**

Wishing you a Smiley Colon!

Show me a patient with Irritable Bowel Syndrome and
I will show you a patient with poorly managed constipation.
Vikas Khurana, MD, MBA
Email:
DrKhurana@SmileyColon.com
Website:
www.SmileyColon.com

Acknowledgements

I would like to thank *Dr. Jamie S. Barkin*, my mentor and a dear friend, who encouraged me to write this book and always supported me to take the road less travelled. My sincere thanks to him for his trust and guidance. I would also like to thank numerous mentors who have shaped my thoughts and investigative styles for years. They're too numerous to enumerate and I humbly bow to them for the wisdom they imparted to me. I am grateful to *Dr. Dinesh Khera* for hours of conversations that clarified my thinking on the book and other matters. I also thank the nurses and the support staff who provided feedback about the concepts.

I will also like to thank the researchers and clinicians who have worked tirelessly to make life better for people suffering with these ailments. I have learnt a great deal from their work and gratefully acknowledge my debt to them.

Thanks to our patients, who have contributed in a fundamental way to the advancement of science by participating in clinical research. I would like to thank my patients who have educated me more than books could and being patient to my seemingly unconventional explanations.

Thanks to *Isha Gulati and Vriti Khurana* for their editorial support and enthusiasm. I thank my wife for her patience and never-ending support whilst I spent hundreds of hours working on this book.

And last, but certainly not least, I thank *my family* for providing guidance and spiritual support at critical times.

The author encourage you to ask questions and find your answers in the "Dr Khurana Replies" section on the website www.SmileyColon.com

Any information on the website www.SmileyColon.com is not to be considered as medical advice. It is only an informational site. Please contact your doctor for your medical needs.

Vikas Khurana, MD can be reached at:

Email:
DrKhurana@SmileyColon.com

Website:
www.SmileyColon.com

www.ingramcontent.com/pod-product-compliance
Lightning Source LLC
Chambersburg PA
CBHW052142270326
41930CB00012B/2993